Blood

Reflections on what unites and divides us

Edited by **Anthony Bale** and **David Feldman**

Pears Institute for the study of Antisemitism
Birkbeck, University of London in collaboration with the Jewish Museum London

Published in Great Britain in 2015 by Shire Publications Ltd (part of Bloomsbury Publishing Plc), PO Box 883, Oxford, OX1 9PL, UK.
PO Box 3985, New York, NY 10185-3985, USA.
E-mail: shire@shirebooks.co.uk   www.shirebooks.co.uk

A CIP catalogue record for this book is available from the British Library.

ISBN: 978 1 78442 138 0
PDF e-book ISBN: 978 1 78442 140 3
ePub ISBN: 978 1 78442 139 7

Gil Anidjar, Anthony Bale, Marc Michael Epstein, David Feldman, Sander Gilman, Robin Judd, Dorothy Porter and Joanne Rosenthal have asserted their right under the Copyright, Designs and Patents Act, 1988, to be identified as the authors of their contributions to this book.

Typeset in Adobe Garamond and ITC Franklin Gothic. Originated by PDQ Digital Media Solutions, Suffolk. Printed in China through Worldprint Ltd.

15 16 17 18 19   10 9 8 7 6 5 4 3 2 1

Shire Publications supports the Woodland Trust, the UK's leading woodland conservation charity. Between 2014 and 2018 our donations will be spent on their Centenary Woods project in the UK.

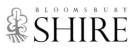

BLOOMSBURY
SHIRE

The cover image is derived from a medieval illustration of a 'wound man', Germany *c.* 1420–30, held by the Wellcome Library, London. The full illustration can be seen on page 23.

Contents

Acknowledgements

This volume of essays has been compiled to complement the exhibition *Blood* at the Jewish Museum London. We are grateful to Abigail Morris, the staff of the Museum and especially to Joanne Rosenthal for the knowledge, skill and enthusiasm they have brought to this collaborative venture.

We would also like to record our thanks to the Birkbeck/Wellcome Trust Institutional Strategic Support Fund for Public Engagement, which made a grant to facilitate this publication.

Dr Jan Davison has managed this project from beginning to end. Her expertise and input have been invaluable.

> Therefore, as I live, saith the Lord GOD, I will prepare thee unto blood, and blood shall pursue thee; surely thou hast hated thine own blood, therefore blood shall pursue thee.

לָכֵן חַי-אָנִי, נְאֻם אֲדֹנָי יְהוִה, כִּי-לְדָם אֶעֶשְׂךָ, וְדָם יִרְדְּפֶךָ; אִם-לֹא דָם שָׂנֵאתָ, וְדָם יִרְדְּפֶךָ

Ezekiel 35:6

This cursed Jew hym hente, and heeld hym faste,
And kitte his throte, and in a pit hym caste.
I seye that in a wardrobe they hym threwe
Where as thise Jewes purgen hire entraille!
O cursed folk of Herodes al newe,
What may youre yvel entente yow availle?
Mordre wol out, certeyn, it wol nat faille,
And namely ther th'onour of God shal sprede;
The blood out crieth on youre cursed dede.

Geoffrey Chaucer, The Prioress's Tale from *The Canterbury Tales*
(late fourteenth century)

No man will treat with indifference the principle of race. It is the key to history and why history is so often confused is that it has been written by men who were ignorant of this principle and all the knowledge it involves… Language and religion do not make a race – there is only one thing which makes a race, and that is blood.

Benjamin Disraeli, *Endymion* (1880)

Blood is a very special juice.

Mephistopheles, in Johann Wolfgang von Goethe, *Faust Part 1* (1808)

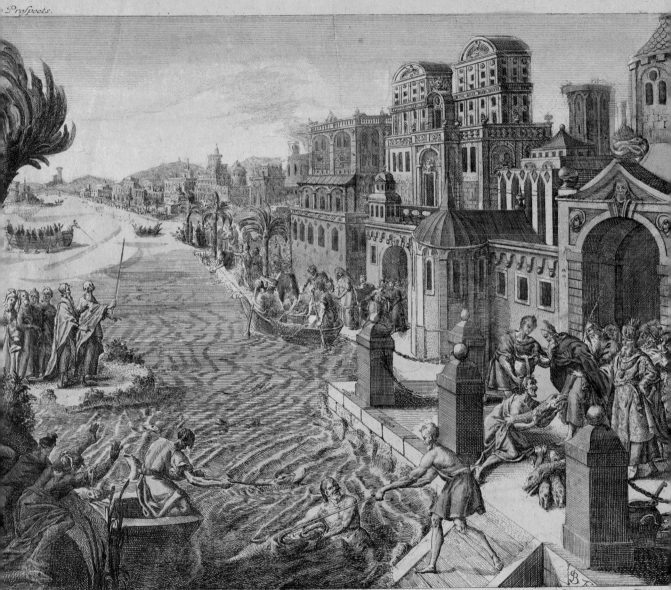

e Plage in Egyptenland, oder die Verwand-
lung alles Waſſers in Blut.

ron thaten, wie Ihnen der Herr gebotten hatte u. hub den Stab auf, und
er, das im Strom war, vor Pharao u. ſeine Knechten u. alles Waſſer in
n Blut verwandelt, u. die Fiſche im Strom ſturben, und der Strom
nd daß die Egyptier nicht trincken konten, des Waſſers aus dem
rd Blut in ganz Egyptenland ſieben Tag lang. 2. B. Moſe Cap. 7. v. 19. 20. 25.

La premiere Plaie en Egyp
Moyse donc et Aaron firent selon que l'Eternel avait c
aiant levé la verge, en frappa les eaux du fleuve. Phar
le voiant, et toutes les eaux du fleuve furent changées
poiſſon qui etoit au fleuve moirut, et le fleuve en a
ment, que les Egyptiens ne pouvoient point boire du
et il y eut du sang par tout le pais d'Egypte Sept
Exode Cap. 7. v. 20. 21. 25.

Se vend à Augsbourg au Negoce en cormei de l'Academia Imperiale des Arts liberaux avec Privilege de Sa Majesté Imperiale et avec Defense ni d'enfaire ni de vendre les Copies.

Introduction

'If you prick us, do we not bleed?'

Shylock, in William Shakespeare, *The Merchant of Venice*, c. 1596.

Blood is something that all humans share: a vital force that courses through our veins – the giver of life. This is the definition of blood at its simplest and most elemental. Look to religious, early medical, racial and historical texts and images and blood takes on other meanings which proliferate in an amazing variety of institutional and cultural contexts. Blood, it transpires, is never simple: blood can always be interpreted.

This book gathers together a range of reflections on how blood, in its regulation and its representation, has been understood as a part of Jewish ritual and culture and how it has been traded as a symbol between Jews and non-Jews and, in particular, between Christians and Jews. Blood is central to Jewish religion and ritual: it has been used by Jews for their own self-definition and yet it has also been used by others to mark Jews' bodies and desires as different. Blood has often had negative connotations, as the Jews' uses of blood – perceived and imagined – have been a staple of antisemitic imagery. Using sources from across the world and from a wide expanse of history, from the biblical past to the present day, these essays present a provocative and rich exploration of how blood can unite and divide.

The essays in this book arise from the exhibition *Blood*, at the Jewish Museum London (November 2015–February 2016), which was conceived in collaboration

The first plague in Egypt, rivers turned to blood (Exodus 7:19). Coloured etching, 1775–79. Wellcome Library, London.

with the Pears Institute for the study of Antisemitism, Birkbeck, University of London. Both the exhibition and the essays present a discontinuous cultural history of blood. We have not tried to provide a comprehensive account: this would be an impossibly large undertaking. Instead, we have focused on the instability of blood, its contentious meanings, and its myriad representations.

The essays presented here are by scholars from a range of fields – history, literature, art history, religious studies and medical humanities – but they are written for a broad audience. The essays cover some of the most difficult issues concerning blood: the rite of circumcision, the outrageous slander of the blood libel, the notion of the Jewish 'race', dreams of conversion, and the boundaries of the body. We provide few answers. Rather, we hope to provoke thoughtful responses to the paradox of blood. Human blood looks the same when one cuts the veins. Yet despite its encompassing universality, the differences ascribed to blood and invested in it have also been central to the idea of the human for thousands of years.

Readers are encouraged to join the debate, and share their own reflections on the meaning of blood, via our dedicated Facebook page and Twitter feed. For further details see **www.jewishmuseum.org.uk/blood**

Anthony Bale
David Feldman
Joanne Rosenthal

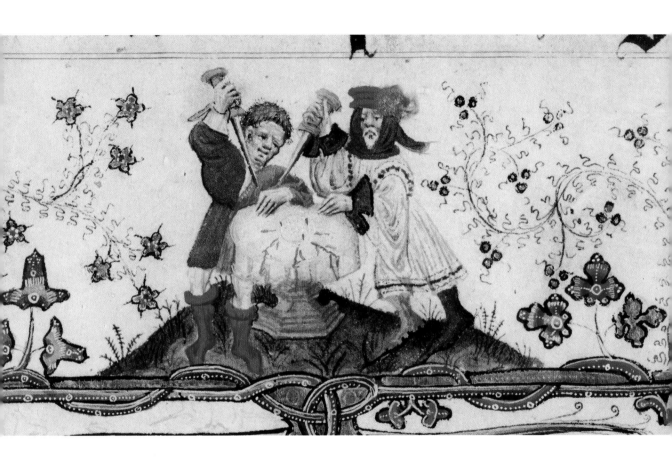

Two men, usually identified as Jews, stab the bread of the Eucharist, which then bleeds. From the Lovell Lectionary, *c*. 1408, England, probably Glastonbury.
©The British Library Board, Harley Ms. 7026 f.13.

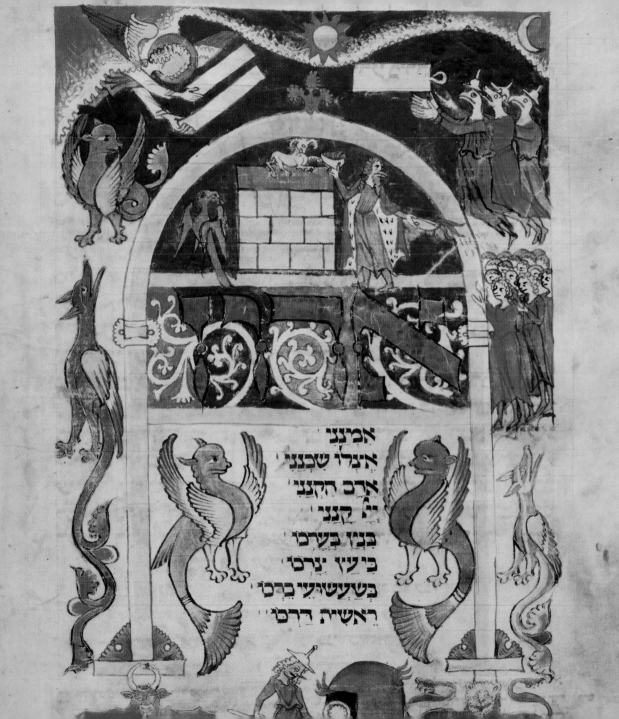

אמצנו
אונזלו שכנצי
אדכ הקבצי
יג קבצי
כבן בערכו
כי צין יצרכו
בשעטשעי ברכו
ראשיה הרכו

In our Veins
Marc Michael Epstein

When we hear the words 'atoning blood' or 'washed in the blood of the Lamb' or 'this is my blood', it is inevitable that we hear them in a Christian voice, through Christian liturgy, situated in Christian culture. But in truth, as both substance and symbol, blood is fundamentally and intrinsically central to Jewish consciousness.

There is a range of meanings for blood in Christian culture, but it is primarily salvific, redeeming – not any blood, mind you, but only the blood of Christ – and essentially metaphoric (mystics and visionaries may be baptized in the blood of Christ, ordinary Christians are baptized in water). Its non-metaphoric reflections tend to be more gruesome – either reflecting the early persecution of Christians (the blood of the martyrs), or the later persecutions of others by Christians (the blood reaching the knees of the horses as the Crusaders slew Muslims in the precincts of the *Haram es Sharif* – the Noble Sanctuary, the Temple Mount).

Jewish culture, which never gave up the idea of literal sacrifice – whether in the form of historical memory or anticipated restoration – conjures for blood at least as broad a range of meanings as it has in Christian culture – if not broader. The Hebrew Bible

The giving of the Law, with Moses sprinkling the blood of the Covenant over the Israelites, depicted in the Hebrew prayer book, Laud Mahzor (Germany, late thirteenth century).
'And Moses took the blood, and sprinkled it on the people, and said: "Behold the blood of the covenant, which the LORD hath made with you in agreement with all these words."'

'וַיִּקַּח מֹשֶׁה אֶת-הַדָּם, וַיִּזְרֹק עַל-הָעָם; וַיֹּאמֶר, הִנֵּה דַם-הַבְּרִית אֲשֶׁר כָּרַת יְהוָה עִמָּכֶם, עַל כָּל-הַדְּבָרִים, הָאֵלֶּה.'

Exodus 24:8
The Bodleian Libraries, University of Oxford, Ms. Laud. Or. 321, folio 127v.

is full of blood. There is the blood of one's brother – that of the first murder, which also stands in for the blood of suffering that should not be ignored. There is the blood to be exacted as penalty for murder. There is the blood of circumcision of sons – shed willingly by Abraham, but neglected by Moses, whose wife Zipporah must swoop in at the last possible moment and accomplish the thankless task, after which she proclaims Moses to be her 'bridegroom of blood.' There is the blood of deception – the kid slain by Joseph's brothers in pretence to their father of Joseph's having been devoured by a wild beast. One of the wonders that God enacts through Moses is the transformation of the waters of the Nile into blood. Although we are told explicitly that this is a 'sign' – that it has a clear symbolic meaning, the precise meaning is unclear: if it is meant as a measure-for-measure judgement upon Pharaoh for destroying the male Israelite newborns, the problem is that he accomplished this by drowning them – no literal blood was shed. The rabbis 'solve' this ambiguity by recounting that Pharaoh also bathed in the blood of Israelite children to cure his leprosy.

Sacrificial blood is extremely varied. The blood of the Passover Sacrifice is displayed on the doorposts of Israelite homes in Egypt as a grand performance of religious defiance in prelude to the departure of God's people from their enslavement. Since the lamb was a baby ram, symbol of the chief Egyptian god, the act of killing it in public during prime time, and spreading its blood all over the front of one's house was analogous to grabbing the likeness of the infant Jesus from the crib on Christmas Eve and running back and forth over its little body on one's driveway in an SUV. The blood of the Covenant is sprinkled on the altar in the Tabernacle. Sprinkled likewise on the sons of Aaron, the blood consecrates the priests of Aaron's line. The blood of the various sacrifices, as well as the blood of any slaughtered animal may not, however, be consumed, for as Leviticus tells us, 'the life of all flesh is its blood.'

Blood is Janus-faced – it can cut (if you will forgive the metaphor) two ways: there is the blood of virgins – the blood of first intercourse – which is celebrated, yet which renders the bride impure. There is the blood of parturition and the blood of menstrual impurity, both tokens of life-giving, yet likewise generators of impurity. There is the blood of the innocent shed by murder, and the blood avenger, who avenges such a murder. There is the blood of enemies in battle, and the avenged blood of God's servants, slain by those enemies. Blood is simultaneously the life force of all beings and a pollutant, powerful and forbidden, holy and impure, to be celebrated and to be avoided. There are very few other substances that are polyvalent or that send such mixed messages. The rabbis, for instance, identify the blood of martyrs as the blood that brings about redemption, eliding it with the blood of sacrifice. The rabbis speak of the blood of the martyrs staining God's porphyrion (purple cloak). But why is God's garment purple anyway? It has, they tell us, been stained by God's trampling of the enemy – of Edom – as one might press the grapes in a winepress. What is it, then, that colours God's garment? The blood of God's saints or of God's foes? It seems to be both at the same time, blood co-mingled with blood.

Ezekiel utilizes the strange metaphor of describing the Israelites as an abandoned girl child wallowing in the blood of birth, who is pitied and nurtured by God and later – when her 'time for love had arrived' – is visited by God as lover. God washes the blood of menstruation from her and enters into a marriage covenant with her, bedecking her in finery. God's hopeful declaration, 'Live in spite of your [parturitive] blood, live in spite of your [menstrual] blood!' refers to the impure state of the (female-generated) 'bloods' of birth and menstruation as an impediment that Israel will overcome. The statement is transformed by the rabbis into an androcentric and even more definitively positive declaration when they assert that the two 'bloods' referred to here are the blood of circumcision and the blood of the Passover sacrifice, which are both pure and male – which is no coincidence. The tenor of God's declaration shifts, and in their reading God promises, even more optimistically, that 'by means of your [circumcisional] blood you shall live, by means of your [Paschal] blood you shall live!' This is a prime example of the ambiguity of blood and its potential uses – here, as a gendered metaphor.

Blood is answered by blood also in an historical frame: Jews in Spain after 1492, who had converted to Christianity in order to avoid losing all their property and possessions, were subjected to a two-tier system in the social network of post-Expulsion Iberian society: there were privileged Old Christians, and New (recently converted) Christians, who experienced discrimination because their blood was not 'pure'. This mindset of *limpieza de sangre* (purity of blood) infected some of their descendants in the Sephardic diaspora, when, returning to Judaism outside of Iberia, they desired to maintain the boundaries of their 'pure' Sephardic communities.

Reflecting this polyvalency, blood is explicitly represented in a number of iconographic contexts within Jewish visual culture. One might point, among very many examples, to the case of the blood flowing from the neck of the Passover Sacrifice in the Griffins' Head Haggadah (Germany, Upper Rhine, *c.* 1310, Jerusalem, the Israel Museum, MS 180/57), the sprinkling of blood on the first Israelite priests during their consecration in the Laud Mahzor, to Pharaoh's bathing in blood in the Mantua Haggadah and contemporary manuscripts. One might marvel over the explicitness of the scenes of bloody martyrdom in the Hamburg Miscellany (Germany, possibly Mainz, *c.* 1427, Hamburg, Staats- und Universitätsbibliothek, MS Cod. Hebr. 37), or discern the apophasis of blood in images of Ezekiel's 'naked and bare' Israel in various manuscript and printed haggadot (as, for example, in the ones illustrated by

Joel ben Simeon, Italy, late fifteenth century, Jerusalem, National Library of Israel, MS Heb. 4° 6130, fols. 9b–10a, and the Prague Haggadah of 1526), or in the surprisingly explicit depictions of women using the *mikveh*, or ritual bath, in a variety of early modern manuscripts of women's prayers and observances (see, for instance, the *Seder Berakhot* (Women's Prayer Book), Vienna, 1736, New York, Library of the Jewish Theological Seminary, MS 4789, fol. 16r).

Is blood beautiful or disgusting? When the rabbis tell us that 'one who has not seen the building of Herod [Herod's improvements to the Second Temple] has never seen a beautiful construction, for it was made of blue and white marble and sparkled like waves in the sea,' we think we understand their aesthetic. But the same rabbis also declared, 'one who has not seen the blood of the sacrifices up to the calves of the priests has never seen a beautiful sight.' Their aesthetic is not necessarily our aesthetic. But one doesn't need to feel that blood is beautiful to know that it is profound, and that it is profoundly '*bon à penser* – good to think with' as the anthropologist Claude Lévi-Strauss put it. Whether the blood is visible or implied, it is with us – it flows in the veins, so to speak, of our culture and our art, makes us live – it is the life of all flesh.

FURTHER READING

- David Biale, ***Blood and Belief*** (University of California Press, 2008)
- Bettina Bildhauer, ***Medieval Blood*** (University of Wales Press, 2010)
- Mitchell Hart (ed.), ***Jewish Blood: Reality and metaphor in history, religion and culture*** (Routledge, 2013)
- Caroline Walker Bynum, ***Wonderful Blood: Theology and Practice in Late Medieval Northern Germany and Beyond*** (University of Pennsylvania Press, 2007)

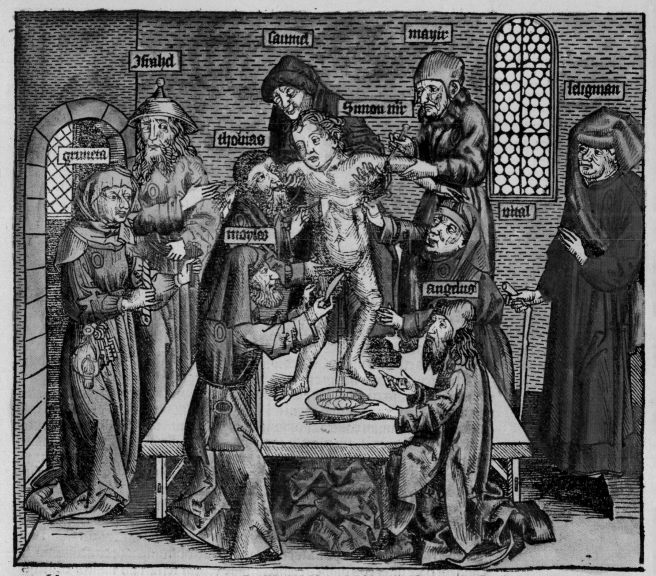

O ſimile etiã ſcelꝰ apꝺ motã oppidũ qꝺ ē ĩ finibꝰ agrí foꝛi iulij pꝰ ꝗnꝗnꝗniũ iudeꝛ pegeꝛt. Nã etiã alị
um pueꝛũ ſiłi mõ mactaueꝛũt. p ꝗ tres eoꝛ captiui venetijs miſſi fueꝛt ꞇ atroci ſupplicꞽo ꝯcremati ſł.
Iterum thurchi inferꝛoꝛem ingreſſi miſiam magna cede ſternunꝛ. Debinc magnã genuenſium vꝛbẽ ca
lpham quã ad meotidem adhuc poſſidebant. Genuenſes eꝛpugnant. ciuitas populoſa ꞇ mercatoꝛibus
plurimũ apta fuit hoc anno ciue genueoſi eã pꝛodente in turchoꝛ niãn. ꝺeuenit in littoꝛe euꝛini maris ſita.

Shylock's Blood
Anthony Bale

In William Shakespeare's troubling and clever play *The Merchant of Venice* (*c.* 1596–7), Bassanio (a Venetian Christian) needs money to pursue the affections of a wealthy local lady, Portia. Bassanio's intimate companion, Antonio (the Venetian merchant of the play's title), borrows 3,000 ducats from Shylock the Jew, secured on the interest of 'a pound of flesh'. When Antonio's ships are reported to have been lost at sea, Shylock demands the return of his bond. But Portia, who has fallen for Bassanio, appears; disguised as a lawyer, and in a brilliant twist, she tells Shylock that he is entitled to his pound of flesh, but that he must not spill a drop of Antonio's blood:

> *This bond doth give thee here no jot of blood;*
> *The words expressly are 'a pound of flesh:'*
> *Take then thy bond, take thou thy pound of flesh;*
> *But, in the cutting it, if thou dost shed*
> *One drop of Christian blood, thy lands and goods*
> *Are, by the laws of Venice, confiscate*
> *Unto the state of Venice.*

The impossibility of the bond saves Antonio, and further humiliates Shylock, whose daughter, Jessica, will later elope with the Christian Lorenzo and convert to his faith.

The martyr's blood: the torture and martyrdom by Jews of Simon of Trent (Simonino di Trento), said to have been martyred in 1475. Woodcut from Hartmann Schedel's *Weltchronik* (Nuremberg, 1493). Cambridge University Library: Inc.0.A.7.2[888], 254v. Reproduced by kind permission of the Syndics of Cambridge University Library.

Tellingly, Portia insists here on 'Christian blood', highlighting Shylock's Jewishness and implying a difference between Christian and Jewish blood. Portia's speech also invokes ancient ideas of the Jews' lust for Christian blood, and this is highlighted when Bassanio says, of the letter that informs him that Antonio's ships are lost: 'The paper [is] as the body of my friend,/ And every word in it a gaping wound,/ Issuing life-blood.' The Christians see the deal they have made with Shylock as a drain on their 'life-blood', the blood of vitality and health.

In many ways, *The Merchant of Venice* is about the meaning of blood and its relation to a person's identity; as Shylock says of Jessica, 'my daughter is my flesh and blood', and Jessica says of Shylock 'I am a daughter to his blood.' We often talk today about our families in terms of 'blood relations', of being 'of the same blood', 'related by blood', as if to suggest that it is in our blood that bonds of family are carried. These figures of speech have been bequeathed to us from the medieval and early modern periods.

Medieval and early modern medicine held that blood contributes to every part of the animal and that, in a healthy person, blood draws off diseases via the veins. Following the important medical theories put forward by Isidore of Seville (d. 636), conventional medical knowledge said that a man's semen was made of the 'foam' of his blood. So it was held that 'blood' was passed on through the father and, in the usual course of things, the child was nourished and sustained by his blood. Accordingly, the child was a direct 'blood' descendant of its father. If a child is made from its father's blood, via his semen, it follows that the child's own blood is directly inherited from the father.

The Merchant of Venice suggests that Jewish, Christian, and Muslim blood is differently legible. One of Portia's suitors, the Moor, the Prince of Morocco, challenges her to compare him to a man from the 'northernward' part of the world: 'And let us make incision for your love,/ To prove whose blood is reddest, his or mine.' It is unclear here whether Morocco is suggesting a radical sameness between his blood and that of the pale-skinned northerner, or that his 'hot' blood is redder and hence stronger than the weaker blood of the northerner. Either way, Morocco challenges the audience to look beyond his 'dark' skin colour and think about the blood that flows through his veins. Shakespeare's play discloses a deep anxiety about the differences – or lack of difference – between Christian and non-Christian bodies.

Similarly, one of the Christian characters in the play, Antonio's friend Salarino, says of Shylock and Jessica:

There is more difference between thy flesh and hers than between jet and ivory; more between your bloods than there is between red wine and rhenish.

The 'rhenish' wine (from the Rhineland) is stronger, more potent, than the red wine; the suggestion is that Jessica's blood is stronger and better, more prized, than Shylock's. In this sense the play tries to deal with the issue of conversion of Jews to Christianity – and, possibly, discloses an anxiety about the significant community of *converso* Spanish and Portuguese Jews who had moved to Elizabethan London during Shakespeare's own time.

Blood itself is central to the bond that Shylock makes with Antonio. But as a theme, it appears in perhaps the most powerful (and probably the most famous) speech in the play, when Shylock appeals to the Venetians to consider him as a human being rather than as a Jew:

I am a Jew. Hath not a Jew eyes? hath not a Jew hands, organs, dimensions, senses, affections, passions? fed with the same food, hurt with the same weapons, subject to the same diseases, healed by the same means, warmed and cooled by the same winter and summer, as a Christian is? If you prick us, do we not bleed? if you tickle us, do we not laugh? if you poison us, do we not die? and if you wrong us, shall we not revenge? if we are like you in the rest, we will resemble you in that. If a Jew wrong a Christian, what is his humility? Revenge. If a Christian wrong a Jew, what should his sufferance be by Christian example? Why, revenge.

Shylock's question – 'If you prick us, do we not bleed?' – appeals to a sense of the Jew's humanity at the same time as anticipating violence towards Jews. But it is also an appeal to his Venetian audience to recognize that his blood (and the pain caused by the spilling of his blood) is similar to Antonio's blood. Shylock's speech is radical and troubling because it is his attempt to reveal the sameness, the sharedness, of blood.

Ultimately, however, *The Merchant of Venice* settles for a vision in which blood can be transformed, as Jessica renounces her blood kinship with her father and bodily difference is restated and confirmed. As Antonio predicts early in the play, 'the Hebrew will turn Christian' confirming Shylock's own assertion that Jews and Christians are more alike than different. Jessica's conversion is planned in a pithy speech, central to which is her leaving behind of Shylock's blood:

Alack, what heinous sin is it in me
To be ashamed to be my father's child!
But though I am a daughter to his blood,
I am not to his manners. O Lorenzo,
If thou keep promise, I shall end this strife,
Become a Christian and thy loving wife.

Jessica sees herself saved by what she calls a 'bastard hope' – a hope that she might be illegitimate, of different blood from Shylock, a break in the bloodline. Ultimately, in an ambiguous conclusion, Jessica steals from her father, runs away to Lorenzo, and appears to leave her Judaism and Jewishness behind. In the world of Shakespeare's Venice, at least, the blood line can be broken, through marriage, distance, and conversion.

FURTHER READING

- Janet Adelman, *Blood Relations: Christian and Jew in* **The Merchant of Venice** (University of Chicago Press, 2008)
- Roland Greene, 'Blood', in *Five Words: Critical Semantics in the Age of Shakespeare and Cervantes* (University of Chicago Press, 2013)
- Lisa Lampert, *Gender and Jewish Difference from Paul to Shakespeare* (University of Pennsylvania Press, 2004)

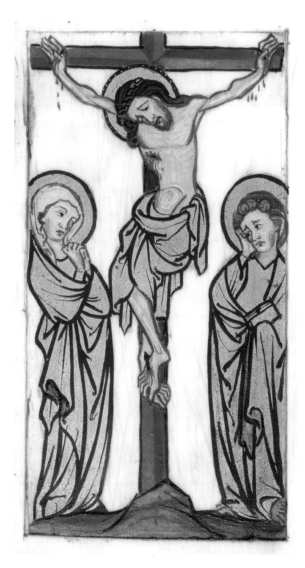

Stigmatic blood: the crucified Christ bleeding from his wounds. In the Middle Ages Jews were increasingly held responsible for Christ's crucifixion. This drew its authority from Matthew 27:25, 'And the whole people answering said, "His blood be upon us and our children."' Devotional booklet, ivory painted with gold, Germany, 1330–50. © Victoria and Albert Museum, London.

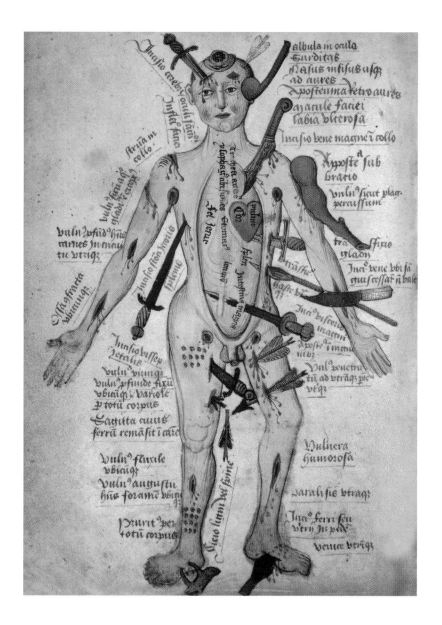

Surgical blood: a medieval German 'wound man', showing wounds and their treatments, from a manuscript of the Apocalypse and other texts, Germany *c.* 1420–30. Wellcome Library, London.

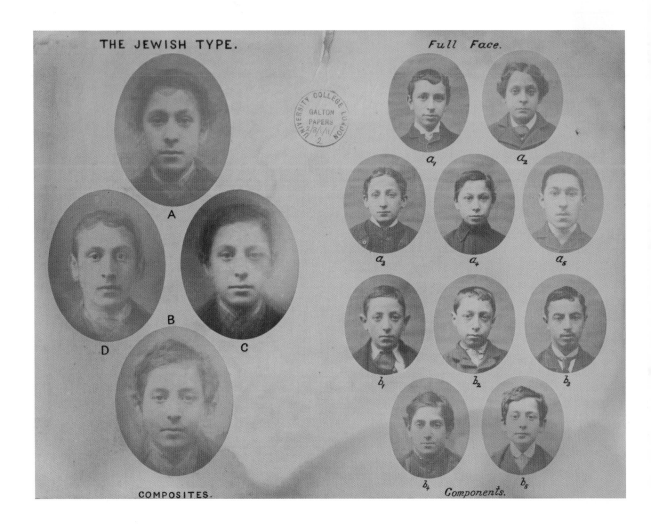

'The Jewish Type', 1885: composite photographs of Jewish boys produced by Francis Galton,
in collaboration with Joseph Jacobs, as part of his research into heredity.
The Galton Papers, UCL Library Services, Special Collections.

Modern Blood
David Feldman

Blood flows in unruly ways. Staunch it here, it surges there.

On 17 August 1840 a correspondent, using the moniker Sigma, wrote to *The Times*:

> *But will it be denied that the religion of the Jews was not essentially a bloody one, and that the altars were reeking not only with the blood of sheep, and goats, and oxen, but that the sanguine stream of human victims also crimsoned the astounded earth, and flowed in propitiation to Jehovah... The very initiation of a Jew was performed in blood (circumcision) forming in this, as in most other matters, so practical an antithesis to the mildness of Christianity where the initiation is by water.*

Sigma's intent was to suggest that the ten Jews in Damascus, who in March of that year had been arrested, tortured, and sentenced to be hanged for the murder of Padre Tomasso, a Capuchin monk, and his servant Ibrahim Amara, might indeed be guilty of the crime. Their alleged motive was the Jews' desire to procure human blood for a Passover ritual. If a Jew really did believe every word of the Old Testament, Sigma suggested, then what might appear to be a crime in the eye of a polished Jewish merchant in London, might not seem so to 'an ignorant and fanatic Jew, in the dead of night, in a by-lane of Damascus.'

Britain in the early nineteenth century was the world's single superpower; it was the forcing house of industrialization, and the apex of modernity. Yet here the blood libel, the accusation that Jews killed Christians to use their blood in rituals, first framed in Norwich in the twelfth century, remained credible to some. Sigma's opinions were not idiosyncratic. The British Consul in Damascus was convinced of the Jews' guilt and *The Times* itself regarded the matter as an open question. Yet 1840 was the last time the blood libel received any widespread credence in Britain.

Five decades later, the Jewish polymath Joseph Jacobs turned to write about one notorious case of blood libel: the disappearance and murder of a boy, Hugh, in Lincoln which had resulted in the judicial execution of eighteen Jews in 1255. Jacobs approached the incident dispassionately, brandishing his credentials as a folklorist. He attributed some blame to the 'injudicious conduct of the Jews in not handing over the body of the lad when they first discovered it.' Here was a measure of how the blood libel had lost all credibility in late nineteenth-century Britain. The Jewish victims' innocence stood so far beyond doubt that their errors could now be owned.

The blood libel supposed not only that Judaism was a religion drenched in blood, but also that the purity of the Jews' blood was a burden to them and that they craved the blood of Christians. Joseph Jacobs, however, was not only a folklorist, he was also a pioneer race scientist. At the same time as he consigned to history both the blood libel and the notion that Jewish blood was inadequate he also vaunted the self-sufficient purity of Jewish blood.

Born in Sydney, Jacobs came to England in 1873 to study at Cambridge University. Two books were formative: Charles Darwin's *The Descent of Man* (1871) and George Eliot's novel *Daniel Deronda* (1876). It is significant that both are intensely concerned with the social and personal consequences of biological inheritance. One objective of *The Descent of Man* was to consider 'the value of the differences between the so-called races of men'. Competition and survival, Darwin claimed, are carried forward by races not by individuals. Eliot's novel addresses a similar issue. It concludes with Daniel's return to the Jewish people, expressed by his marriage to Mirah, and his departure with her for 'the East'. Biology determines Deronda's destiny.

In the 1880s Jacobs collaborated with Francis Galton, Charles Darwin's cousin, who in 1883 coined the term 'eugenics' and was on a quest to trace the influence of heredity on different races and families. Together the two men ventured to the Jews' Free School in Whitechapel to take photographs. Using Galton's technique of composite photography they aimed to arrive at an image of 'the Jewish type'. Jacobs imitated Galton's study of *Hereditary Genius* with his account of 'Jewish ability', he took note of the size and shape of skulls and in 1885 delivered a paper on 'The racial characteristics of modern Jews' to the luminaries of the Anthropological Institute.

Blood was race in the vernacular. In his last novel, *Endymion*, published in 1880, Benjamin Disraeli set forward that 'No man will treat with indifference the principle of race. It is the key to history and … there is only one thing which makes a race, and that is blood.' And the same principle had been used against Disraeli by his enemies. According to one, he was 'English neither in blood nor in sympathy.' Inevitably, as Jacobs and others strived to convey heredity to a broad reading public they reached, casually it seems, for the sanguinary metaphor of descent. Presenting his research into Jewish intellect, Jacobs explained, 'The names of those who are Jews only in blood and not in creed, have an asterisk affixed to them; those of half Jewish blood have an obelisk prefixed.'

Joseph Jacobs claimed that the Jews were, with minor exceptions, a pure race, unified by common descent. Referring to the photographs he had worked on with Galton he wrote: 'In these Jewish composites we have the nearest representations we can hope to possess of the lad Samuel as he ministered before the Ark, or the youthful David when he tended his father's sheep.' He endowed the Jews' racial singularity with a religious significance. This lay in their gift of monotheism and the moral edifice that Jewish civilization built. Conveniently, the significance of Jewish blood was universal as well as particular.

It might be tempting for us to regard the decaying credibility of the blood libel as one symptom of the march of reason but Jacobs' participation in both the burial of blood libel and the birth of race theory should alert us to the fact that the history of ideas is not simply a history of progress. The Damascus Jews were never proven innocent. It was only when their accusers in Damascus and Alexandria were routed and fell from power that the Jews' critics fell silent. It was politics and war that shaped knowledge, not the reverse. And the same can be said for the doctrine of race. This doctrine of blood proved too attractive and too protean to be regulated by a handful of Jewish scholars. Jewish and non-Jewish scientists corrected Jacobs: the Jews, they agreed, were an impure race. It was this very mongrel quality that Nazi race theory seized upon. Here too it was war, not science, which ultimately defeated their bloody project.

FURTHER READING

- John M. Efron, ***Defenders of the Race: Jewish Doctors and Race Science in Fin-de-Siècle Europe*** (Yale University Press, 1994)
- David Feldman, 'Conceiving Difference: Religion, Race and the Jews in Britain, *c.* 1750–1900', in ***History Workshop Journal*** (August 2013)
- Jonathan Frankel, ***The Damascus Affair: "Ritual Murder," Politics, and the Jews in 1840*** (Cambridge University Press, 1997)

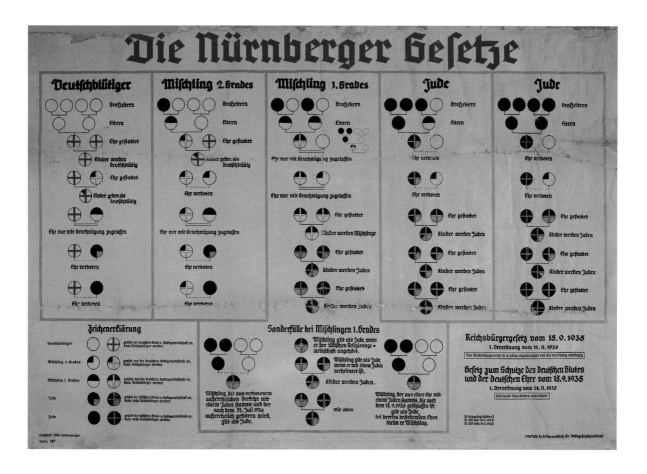

An illustration of how the Nuremberg Laws, 'For the Protection of German Blood and German Honour', were to be implemented. The Laws, passed on 15 September 1935, forbad marriages and sexual relations 'between Jews and nationals of German or kindred blood'. The wording highlights the persistence of 'blood' in Nazi racial thought.
United States Holocaust Memorial Museum Collection, Gift of Virginia Ehrbar through Hillel at Kent State University.

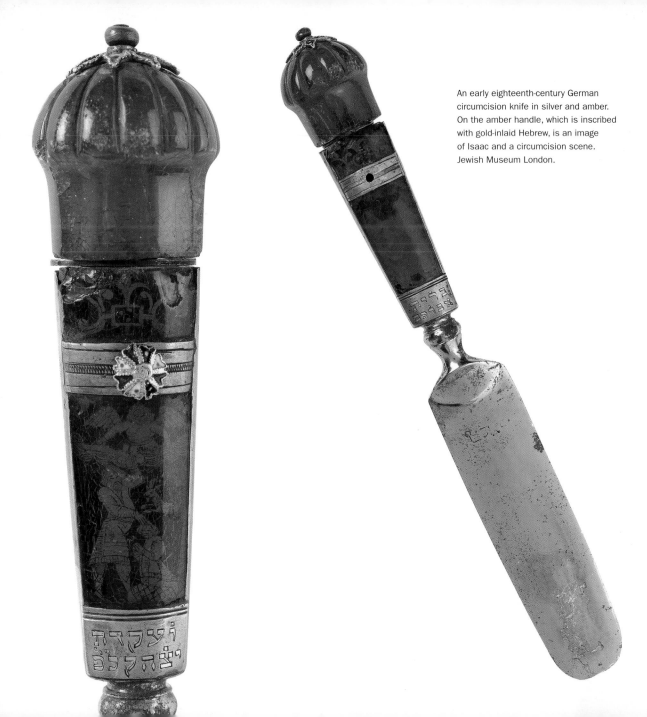

An early eighteenth-century German circumcision knife in silver and amber. On the amber handle, which is inscribed with gold-inlaid Hebrew, is an image of Isaac and a circumcision scene. Jewish Museum London.

Blood Imagery, Jewish Rituals, and Social Activism

Robin Judd

At a May 2013 press forum, the twelve candidates for New York City mayor articulated positions on a surprising subject, *metzitzah b'peh*, the traditional use of oral suction to remove impurities from an infant's wound after circumcision. The rite has long been controversial and modified by many Jews since infants can contract herpes from a *mohel*, or circumciser, when he sucks the blood to 'cleanse' the circumcision wound. Within seconds of the mayoral candidate forum, the blogosphere was replete with accusations concerning Jewish bloodthirstiness. The bloody rite had touched a nerve, but few of those commenting on the supposed relationship between Jews and blood were aware that such a discourse had a long history or that its history was inexorably linked with anxieties about Jewish rites.

Since the early nineteenth century, Jews and non-Jews from different geographical areas and religious, political, and professional orientations have paid attention to the alleged linkages between blood and the Jewish rites of circumcision and kosher butchering (the laws surrounding the slaughter of animals in ways that render the meat kosher). Indeed, the rites are bloody. Each requires a sharp incision and stipulates some kind of blood loss. During kosher butchering, the *shochetim* (slaughterers) are required to drain animals of their blood after they slaughter the animal.

At a circumcision, the *mohel* must shed at least two drops of the child's blood (even if the child is born without a foreskin) and use suction to rid the wound of excess blood. Yet, when relying on blood imagery to make sense of Jewish rituals, those commenting on the rites have invoked – and continue to summon – matters seemingly tangential to the rite itself: concerns about the meaning and limits of religious toleration, cultural anxieties about sexuality, and medical concerns about public health and disease.

Blood mattered in the late nineteenth- and twentieth-century European imagination of Jewish rituals and it continues to be salient today. Discussions about Jewish rites raised concerns about blood in at least three different ways. First, critics suggested that the alleged blood centeredness of the rites demonstrated (or demonstrates) Jewish cruelty. In describing kosher butchering as a rite in which 'torrents of blood' allegedly pour from the animal's neck or by emphasizing a life-threatening 'bloody wound' of circumcision, observers let hover the inference that not only were Jewish rituals brutal, but that Jews were cruel as well. This linkage of blood and rite even found its way into literature and film. Consider how Thomas Mann depicted kosher butchering in *The Magic Mountain* (1924). His protagonist, Leo Naphta, was the son of a *shohet*. As a youngster, Naphta observed his father elatedly 'catch the spurting steaming blood' of the animals he slaughtered.

Second, deeply influenced by changing discourses of public health, medicalization, religious toleration, and governmental jurisdiction, observers of Jewish rites questioned whether the blood of circumcision or kosher butchering served as some kind of contaminant. Opponents of kosher butchering, for example, often portrayed the blood on the abattoir floor as posing a danger to other animals and butchers. Worried that the blood could spread tuberculosis (TB) or other epidemics to the abattoir population or local residents, they drew from an odd fusion of biology, bacteriology,

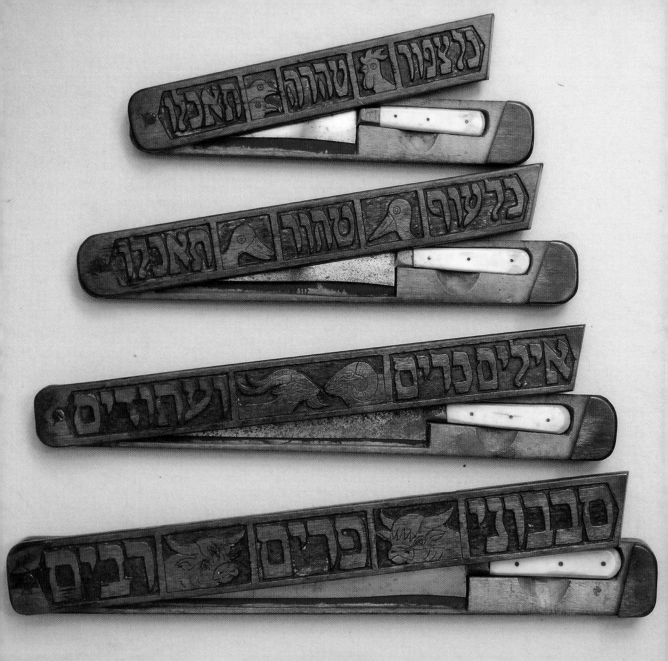

Shechita knives for the slaughter of animals according to Jewish law. The procedure consists of a rapid incision which severs the major structures, arteries and veins in the neck, killing the animal and draining its blood.
The Gross Family Collection Trust.

eugenics, and social Darwinism to link the blood of butchered animals with the illnesses typically associated with urbanization and moral deviancy. Circumcision opponents, too, linked the rite of *metzitzah b'peh* with hepatitis, tuberculosis and gonorrhoea. Especially after the 1890s, when a glass tube had become available for oral suction and when a series of syphilis cases had been publicized, many worried that *mohelim* could spread sexual infections if they practised the traditional form of *metzitzah b'peh*. Several contemporary hepatitis cases have been linked to *metsitah b'peh*, the issue that prompted the question at the 2013 mayoral forum, and contemporary critics have warned that *metzitzah b'peh* could lead to uncontrollable plagues of epidemics.

Third, possibly influenced by discourses concerning vampirism and deviancy, some critics described Jewish rites and their practitioners as blood drinking and charged that Jews not only drank blood but that they gained a profit from it. During the first half of the twentieth century, for example, several Central European states promulgated laws forbidding Jews from ingesting the blood of slaughtered animals or selling the slaughtered animals' blood. Late-nineteenth and early twentieth-century writers penned antisemitic tracts describing blood-drinking *mohelim* who used the infants' blood for *matzah* or kosher wine. Given the interest in the alleged blood-thirst of Jewish rites, it was not surprising that some nineteenth- and twentieth-century actors conflated Jewish rituals with the increasingly popular charge, usually called blood libel, that Jews used the blood of non-Jews for Jewish ritualistic purposes. Imagining the *mohel* or *shohet* as a murderer, critics looked to blood libel to affirm Jewish rituals' brutality and Jewish rituals as proof of the blood libel's existence. Townspeople and local officials often blamed local ritual practitioners when blood libel charges were made. Such antisemitic imagery was not limited to the nineteenth century. A twentieth-century comic book, for example, featured a monstrous-looking *mohel* for whom *metzitzah b'peh* is described as 'delicious' and 'icing on the cake.'

As the mayoral forum suggests, the attempts to link Jewish rites with blood are part of larger patterns and processes of history. When invoking blood imagery to depict Jewish rites, detractors unknowingly repeat the historical complaints that had been uttered by their predecessors. Critics have – and this continues – censured Jewish rites for being at best medically neutral and at worst dangerous. They worry that the rites pose an unnecessary social and political barrier between Jews and non-Jews. Proponents also repeat past arguments. In looking to blood imagery, they champion Jewish rites as prophylaxes, which create no hindrance to Jewish social or political integration. Both look to the connections between rituals and blood as a way to make sense of the world in which they live.

FURTHER READING

- David Biale, ***Blood And Belief: The Circulation of a Symbol Between Jews and Christians*** (University of California Press, 2007)
- John Efron, ***Medicine and the German Jews: A History*** (Yale University Press, 2001)
- Robin Judd, ***Contested Rituals: Circumcision, Kosher Butchering, and Jewish Political Life in Germany, 1843–1933*** (Cornell University Press, 2007)
- Elizabeth Wyner Mark (ed.), ***The Covenant of Circumcision: New Perspectives on an Ancient Jewish Rite*** (Brandeis University Press, 2003)

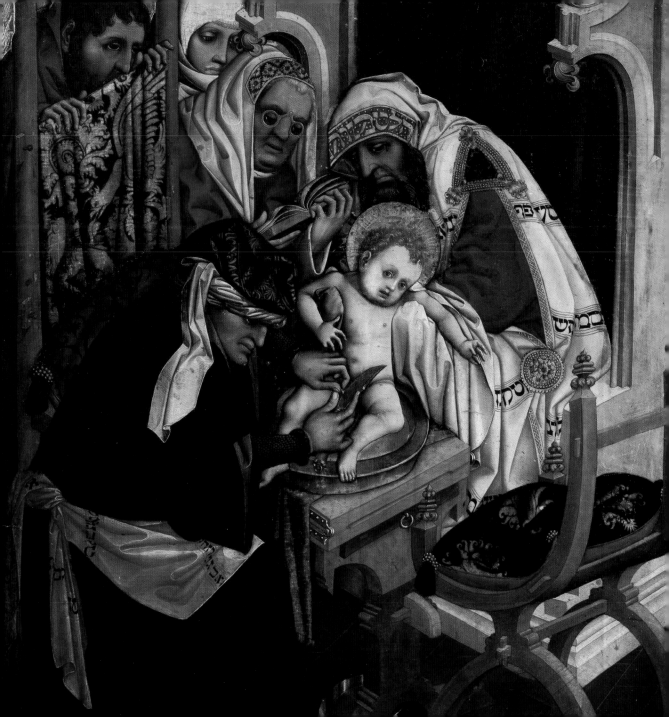

Sucking Blood

Sander L. Gilman

Ritual practice defines religion, whether it is the Christmas tree of Prince Albert or the even more ancient practice of infant male circumcision undertaken by Jews and Muslims. But ritual practice is always assumed to be unchanging, because it is seen as fundamental. However, today's Jewish-Christian 'Hanukkah bush', commonplace in the United States, would have been unimaginable to the Victorians and we know that the ritual circumcision of Jewish boys is different today than it was at the time Albert introduced the Christmas tree into Victorian England in 1840.

In the mid-nineteenth century, Jews in the German states created the Society for the Friends of Reform in Frankfurt in 1843. Drawing on Enlightenment ideas of a division between public practice and personal belief, this group claimed that religious circumcision of male infants, the *brit milah*, was unnecessary as it was neither a religious obligation nor a symbolic act. This was in direct response to the finding of the Frankfurt Public Health Authority on 8 February 1843 that circumcision had to be carried out under medical supervision as it was seen as placing infants at risk. With the expanding role of medicine in the nineteenth century came further opposition; certain aspects of the traditional practice of Jewish circumcision such as the *metzitzah b'peh*, which requires the *mohel* (ritual circumcisor) to orally suck blood from the wound immediately following the excision of the foreskin, were deemed unhygienic. Outbreaks of syphilis and tuberculosis from 1805 to 1865

The Circumcision of Christ by Jewish priests, from the Tucher Altarpiece (Nuremberg c. 1440–50). Suermondt-Ludwig-Museum, Aachen; photo: Anne Gold, Aachen.

were blamed on *mohelim*. Many reformers who wished to keep circumcision as a Jewish practice thus advocated *metzitzah* be performed using a sponge or a glass tube. As a result of such debates acculturated Jews in Central and Western Europe practised circumcision less and less; and if it was undertaken it increasingly followed the new hygienic practice.

In modernity, circumcision in general became a hot topic. An anonymous author stated in a leading German paediatric journal in 1872: 'The circumcision of Jewish children has been widely discussed in the medical press as is warranted with topics of such importance. But it is usually discussed without the necessary attention to details and the neutrality that it deserves. Indeed, it has not been free of fanatic anti-Semitism.' But Jewish reformers countered such antisemitic interpretations, arguing that God's laws concerning blood, whether in the act of circumcision or ritual slaughter, were a sign of His prescient knowledge of hygiene. 'We may go to Moses for instruction in some of the best methods in hygiene,' Sir William Osler, the most famous physician of the early twentieth century, stated in 1914.

In 2012 in New York City, *metzitzah*, which continues to be practised among ultra-Orthodox Jews, was again been blamed for infant deaths, this time from herpes, and the local health department tried to require parental notification of the risks of such procedures. That year about 3,600 male infants were circumcised with direct oral suction. Their risk of contracting herpes was estimated at roughly 1 in 4,000. The Center for Disease Control and Prevention called the procedure unsafe and recommended against it. Every *mohel* was required to collect a consent form from parents advising against oral suction because it 'exposes an infant to the risk of transmission of herpes simplex virus infection, which may result in brain damage or death.' This demand was vociferously opposed by the religious authorities noting that the procedure was not, is not, and can never be the cause of any possible danger to the health of the infant. Yet given that attributions of sexually transmitted infections to this ritual had been made in New York City as early as 1879, such suspicion may well be understood.

The consent forms were virtually *never* used, though some health authorities said they believed that requiring consent did not go far enough. 'It's crazy that we allow this to go on,' said Dr Joel A. Forman, a professor of paediatrics at Mount Sinai School of Medicine (speaking in September 2012). The traditionalists, among them ultra-Orthodox Rabbi William Handler, argued, 'this process is being created without a shred of evidence'. He continued, 'The city is lying, and slandering compassionate rabbis.' A. Romi Cohn, an Orthodox Jew who is head of the American Board of Ritual Circumcision, stated, 'We do it because *Hashem* (God) commands us, and because it's healthy and necessary'. After conducting a *bris*, or circumcision ceremony, in 2015 at a synagogue in Midwood, Brooklyn, Cohn noted, 'Whenever God tells us to do something, it is to our benefit.'

And so blood remains at the centre of such debates even in 2015. On 24 February 2015, officials in the new Democratic administration of New York mayor Bill de Blasio told reporters in a conference call that, under a tentative agreement between the city of New York and ultra-Orthodox rabbis, any *mohelim* suspected of infecting babies with herpes during the circumcision rite will have to undergo DNA testing. It was planned that this innovation would also lead to scrapping parental consent forms for the procedure. If there is a DNA match between the herpes virus in the *mohel* and an infected infant, the *mohel* will be banned from performing *metzitzah* for life.

The *intended consequence* of this change to the legal requirement to inform parents about risk is to expose infants to a procedure that 'may result in brain damage or death' because of the potential risk that the *mohel* will infect the infant. But the *unintended consequence*, unstated and undebated, which has always been present, is the risk to the *mohel* from 'blood-borne pathogens such as hepatitis B, hepatitis C, and HIV which may be transmitted from an asymptomatic but infected neonate [newborn child] to the *mohel*,' as a report from the *Pediatric Infectious Disease Journal* noted in 2000. Blood is necessary to life and to ritual but the shedding of blood is dangerous for all concerned.

FURTHER READING

- Shaye J. D. Cohen, **Why Aren't Jewish Women Circumcised? Gender and Covenant in Judaism** (University of California Press, 2005)
- Sander L. Gilman, 'Decircumcision: The First Aesthetic Surgery,' **Modern Judaism** 17 (1997): 201–11
- Sander L. Gilman, **Image and Illness: Case Studies in the Medical Humanities** (Transaction Publishers, 2015)
- Robin Judd, **Contested Rituals: Circumcision, Kosher Butchering, and Jewish Political Life in Germany, 1843–1933** (Cornell University Press, 2007)
- Eric Kline Silverman, **From Abraham to America: A History of Jewish Circumcision** (Rowman & Littlefield Publishers, 2006)

The account of a Jewish circumcision ceremony, by John Evelyn (1620–1706), an English diarist. Evelyn travelled abroad for four years, and in 1645 visited Rome where he witnessed this circumcision. *Memoirs, Illustrative of the Life and Writings of John Evelyn* (London: Henry Colburn, 1819), I.125.

I went to the Ghetto, where the Jewes dwell as in a suburbe by themselues; being invited by a Jew of my acquaintance to see a Circumcision. I passed by the Piazza Judea, where their Seraglio begins; for, being inviron'd wth walls, they are lock'd up every night. In this place remaines yet part of a stately fabric, which my Jew told me had been a palace of theirs for the ambassador of their nation when their country was subject to the Romans. Being lead through the Synagogue into a privat house, I found a world of people in a chamber: by and by came an old man, who prepared and layd in order divers instruments brought by a little child of about 7 yeares old in a box. These the man layd in a silver bason; the knife was much like a short razor to shut into ye haft. Then they burnt some incense in a censer, wch perfum'd the rome all the while the ceremony was performing. In the basin was a little cap made of white paper like a capuchin's hood, not bigger than the finger; also a paper of a red astringent powder, I suppose of bole; a small instrument of silver, cleft in the middle at one end to take up the prepuce withall; a fine linen cloth wrapped up. These being all in order, the women brought the infant, swaddl'd, out of another chamber, and delivered it to the Rabbie, who carried and presented it before an altar or cupbord dress'd up, on which lay the 5 Bookes of Moses, and the Commandments a little unrowled; before this, with profound reverence, and mumbling a few words, he waved the child to and fro awhile; then he deliver'd it to another Rabbie, who sate all this time upon a table. Whilst the ceremony was performing, all the company fell a singing an Hebrew hymn in a barbarous tone, waving themselves to and fro, a ceremony they observe in all their devotions.

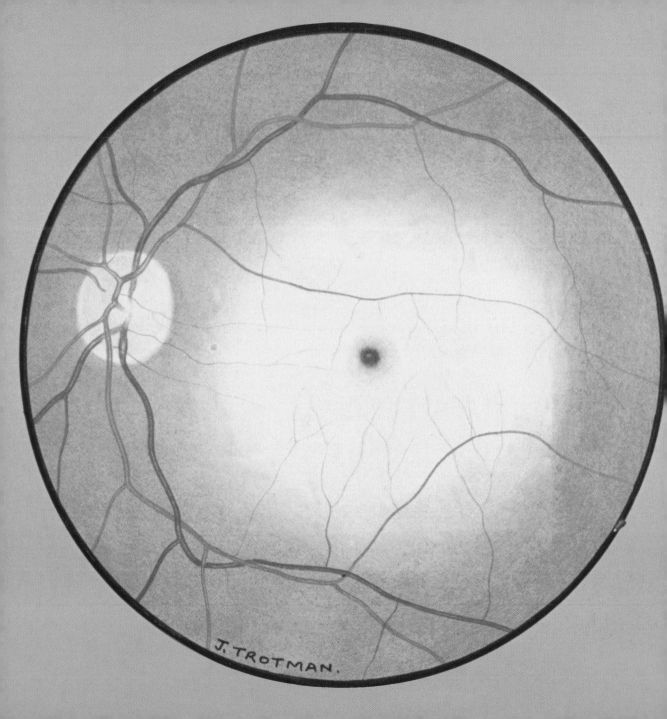

J. TROTMAN.

Blood Archaeology, Disease Prevention, and Eugenic Affirmation

Dorothy Porter

Blood archaeology separates Wizards from Muggles, is the criterion of uniqueness of the Yamato people and linked the German folk to their territory in Richard Walther Darré's Nazi belief in 'Blood and Soil'. Ideas of biological superiority symbolically represented in blood ancestry have motored genocidal politics in historical fact and fiction. Given the politics of the symbolic function of blood ancestry, can the investigation and practical application of knowledge of biological inheritance result in anything other than the reification of scientific racialism and biological normativity? In other words, can the understanding and application of genetic knowledge be differentiated from what Laurie Zoloth, bioethicist at Feinberg School of Medicine, has termed the 'eugenic imperative' even in the cause of disease prevention and alleviating suffering? The significance of these questions is nowhere more forcefully

Image of the retina. The cherry-red spot is an early sign of Tay Sachs disease. Tay Sachs
is a neurodegenerative disorder caused by a genetic mutation which is far more prevalent among
Ashkenazi Jews than within the general population.
Wellcome Images.

highlighted and contested than in the practice of Jewish genetic screening for a range of inheritable diseases which have high frequencies in people of Ashkenazi and Sephardic Jewish descent. Rabbinical and secular Jewish conflict surrounding the ethical status of the organization Dor Yeshorim has exemplified this contest.

In 1985 Rabbi Joseph Ekstein of Brooklyn, New York, set up Chevra Dor Yeshorim (The Association of the Upright Generation) after his fourth child had died of Tay Sachs disease. Tay Sachs is a fatal neurodegenerative disorder that begins in the foetal stage and results in cascading malfunction from the age of six months leading to blindness and convulsions ending in premature death usually before the age of three. It is a recessive mutation on gene 13 and, like sickle cell anaemia and cystic fibrosis, requires both parents to carry it for its expression in offspring. One in 300 people carry the gene in the general population but one in 25 carry it in people of Ashkenazi Jewish descent. Rabbi Ekstein believed the methods of Tay Sachs prevention that involved abortion, artificial insemination or screening of pre-implantations outside the womb were incongruous with halakhic law and thus founded a confidential screening system with the goal of eliminating the disease within the community. Children in Orthodox Jewish high schools and college students were offered screening but only provided with a biological compatibility number rather than the actual results of the test. Couples planning to marry called a 'hotline' to check if their numbers were compatible or not. Ekstein opted for the non-disclosure methodology in order to avoid stigmatization and discrimination that might lead to individuals becoming unmarriageable. This was especially significant for the system of arranged marriages within the Hasidic, ultra-Orthodox community.

The internationally renowned medical ethicist and professor of medicine at Mount Sinai Medical College, Dr Fred Rosner, has praised Dor Yeshorim and fully supports its screening function. 'I think Dor Yeshorim performs a tremendous service … Screening is a wonderful thing to do, and if you can avoid the birth of a potentially lethally affected child, that is a good thing.' Rosner points out that opposition to abortion within Orthodox Judaism means screening is an essential tool for decision-making within the community.

Since the 1980s Dor Yeshorim has added an additional eight fatal degenerative diseases to its screening process. On request, Dor Yeshorim will also screen for Gaucher's disease, which results from the lack of an inheritable enzyme that prevents fatty substances building up and enlarging organs. Ekstein has been accused of 'playing God' by the founder of the Jewish Genetic Disease Consortium, Stuart Ditcheck, for withholding information from individuals who have tested positive for Gaucher's because therapeutic enzyme replacement given to children before they reach their late teens can prevent a lifetime of suffering. Moshe Dovid Tendler, professor of medical ethics at Yeshiva University who teaches Talmudic Law and is a trained microbiologist, has been a longer and even more vocal critic of Dor Yeshorim's non-disclosure. 'The idea that Dor Yeshorim has genetic information and refuses to share it with the person who it belongs to is unfair, irrational, and almost anti-American. If you submit blood, you should be able to have the results,' Tendler claims. And he points out that non-disclosure does not prevent stigmatization, 'When a match is proposed and nothing happens people naturally ask, why didn't this happen? They submitted to Dor Yeshorim and then decided not to get married. This reveals immediately to their entire Jewish community that there are two people who are blemished.'

Objections to non-disclosure have led to other testing centres being established in the United States offering carrier screening and education such as the Center for Jewish Genetics founded in 1997 by a cooperative of Jewish and children's hospital associations in Chicago. It offers screening for 85 genetic disorders including 19 of what it terms 'Jewish Genetic Disorders' resulting from the 'Founder Effect' and genetic drift amongst the Jewish diaspora in Eastern Europe from *c.* 70 CE. While not opposed to genetic testing Tendler nevertheless is concerned with the broader consequences of ever-wider levels of testing: 'The question arises, when do you stop? There are close to 90 genes you wouldn't want to have. Will this lead to people showing each other computer print outs of their genetic conditions? We'll never get married.'

Zoloth's critique of the eugenic imperative of Jewish genetic testing, however, addresses the larger issue of ancestry, disease prevention and scientifically reified racialism and biologistic normalization. Jewish genetic testing dramatically intersects with the hotly disputed legitimacy of using self-identified racial evaluations (SIRES) as ancestry information markers (AIMS) for disease analysis, prevention and therapeutic targeting. On one level debate has focused on the insecure scientific value of racial self-identification reporting. At another, AIMS, or ancestry population genetics, has been identified as a further biologization of the historically constructed categories of race and stereotypes of biological ability and disability. Duana Fullwiley, for example, has argued that asthma research done amongst Hispanic admixture populations since 2005 privileged AIMS over environmental determinants of disease as a form of affirmative action genetic identity politics that unavoidably reifies scientific racialism. Parallel critiques have been forwarded by Disability Activists regarding the biologistic exclusion of human variety through genetic screening for characteristics normatively constructed as pathological.

Comparable arguments have been echoed by Tendler: 'We are affirming eugenics, the idea that Jews are the repository of bad genes …. There should be some sensitivity to the history of eugenics, especially at a time when anti-Semitism is on the increase worldwide.' The willingness of Jews to participate in genetic testing has made them a target for pharmaceutical and biotechnical development research and marketing. Furthermore, the experience of the Jewish community spanning decades of testing has provided an informational and sociological model for reprogenetics as a whole, including the increasing use of pre-implantation genetic diagnosis (PGI) not only for diseases but for characteristics such as eye colour. AIMS analysis extends the capacity of PGI beyond disease prevention to the potential construction of 'better babies' according to politically dominant ideas of the normal and the pathological.

Grounded in the Talmudic morality of the Jewish obligation to the next generation Jewish genetic testing uniquely complicates contemporary debates exploring eugenics in the DNA age. Perhaps, however, as Christine Rosen has pointed out, 'Given the Jewish community's tragic history of … being treated as a people genetically unfit to live' Jewish genetic testing offers unique historical insights not found elsewhere.

FURTHER READING

- Elliott Dorff and Laurie Zoloth (eds.), *Jews and Genes: The Genetic Future in Contemporary Jewish Thought* (The Jewish Publication Society, March 1, 2015)
- Dorothy Porter, 'Darwinian Disease Archeology: Genomic Variants and the Eugenic Debate', *History of Science* 1 (2012): 432–452
- Christine Rosen, 'Eugenics – Sacred and Profane', *The New Atlantis: A Journal of Technology and Society* (2003), Vol. 2: 79–89
- Fred Rosner, 'Jewish Medical Ethics: Genetic Screening and Genetic Therapy', *Jewish Virtual Library* (http://www.jewishvirtuallibrary.org/jsource/Judaism/genetic.html) Last accessed 25 June 2015

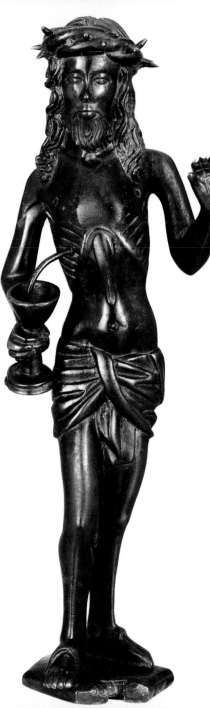

Christ as 'Man of Sorrows', offering blood from
the wound in his side into a Eucharist chalice.
Bronze sculpture (Germany, 1480).
'For this is my blood of the new testament, which
shall be shed for many unto remission of sins.'
Hic est enim sanguis meus novi testamenti,
qui pro multis effundetur in remissionem peccatorum.
Matthew 26:28
© Victoria and Albert Museum, London.

Universal Blood
Gil Anidjar

There is nothing, it seems, more universal than blood. From murder to sacrifice, from menstruation to circulation, our humanity appears to be drenched in blood. So how exactly did blood become Jewish? How did blood move from a universal, 'blood is the life', to a particularly obvious, well, particular, 'Jewish blood'? Someone had to conceive of human beings as being of 'flesh and blood', perhaps of different blood. Someone also had to come up with the idea that blood could define, figure, and bind the community. And who else but the Jews? With their covenant of blood, their blood sacrifices, their concern with menstruation, their (bloodless) dietary restrictions, Jews – or at least the ancient Hebrews – had blood on their mind. And let us not forget Jewish mothers, for it is with them and out of them, is it not, according to the rabbis, that Jewish blood is preserved and transmitted through the generations?

Now, some enlightened minds will no doubt point out that there is no such thing as Jewish blood, not really. It is just a figure, a symbol, a belief, even, one not to be taken literally. Still, who would disagree that Jews have believed in God, I mean, in blood? The angry and avenging God of the Old Testament is certainly remembered for His peculiar brand of blood justice (some give Him the privilege of having invented violence and hatred, since these are apparently and exclusively 'religious' phenomena). Don't we agree, at the very least, that blood is not a Greek concern? Did not the Greeks invent politics out of (and away from) tribal blood? Did they not invent justice to break with blood-murder and revenge? And yet blood fills the dactylic hexameter of Homer. Among his many blood-related activities, Odysseus famously provides a blood fix to the hankering souls of Hades. Empedocles came pretty close to saying 'everything is blood', and Aristotle is (incorrectly) remembered as the haematocentric philosopher-physician *par excellence*. So perhaps blood is universal after all (as universal, that is, as Athens and Jerusalem). But what, then, of Jewish blood? Besides, when was the last time you went to see an exhibition on Greek blood? Blood almost sounds Jewish. This brings us back to the question of community, to the community of blood, and to the individual as 'flesh and blood'. Jewish flesh and blood too?

It may come as a surprise but the phrase 'flesh and blood' never appears in the Old Testament. That is just not the way the Bible thinks. Remember what Adam says when introduced to his former rib? 'This at last is bone of my bones and flesh of my flesh', a phrasing that has made its way into Jewish marriage rituals. Similarly, the notion that 'blood is the life' is actually a mistranslation that substitutes 'life' for 'soul' (*nefesh*, *anima*). Same difference, you might say: life and soul, blood or bone. But consider that this notion of a community of bones is a powerful one, which puts temporal and spatial limits to that which is shared by family and kin (groupings that the Bible would never imagine as 'blood'). The blood of generations, lineage as blood, simply does not exist in the Hebrew Bible. It was Paul, first name Saint, who started bending things in that direction and elaborated a theology of blood, Christ's blood.

By the Middle Ages, Christians were informed that, following an admittedly strange assertion made in the New Testament ('*Hoc est corpus meum*'), they had to drink the blood of Christ and eat his flesh (see? flesh and blood!). They had to do it regularly, if not consistently, for that was the way to integrate 'the mystical body of Christ' (in other words the Church, the community of blood). It quickly became evident to those Christians that their blood was special. Pure as the white snow, or rather, pure as Jesus' blood. The purity of blood – an interesting idea that was bound to all kinds of great developments. First, *noblesse oblige*. The budding aristocracy started to rethink notions of lineage along the lines of blood. They were assisted by the reactivation of Roman notions of *consanguinitas* (we won't get into the mistranslations at work there), the reception of Aristotle's haematocentric embryology (misunderstood? you betcha!), and by a lineage that was increasingly affected by a Christological, and haematological, zeitgeist.

Christians were becoming the first community of blood. Interestingly enough, they also became sensitive to the safety and security of their blood (later their descendants would invent the notion of 'blood banks'). This makes sense, if you think about it. If their blood was indeed different and special, why would those lacking it not come after them, or at least after their children? The blood libel finds one of its powerful origins in this new configuration (and so does Dracula). By the same token, other communities were recast as communities of (impure) blood, for only those who drank the blood of Christ had a claim on the purity of blood. And it would have to stay that way. That is why *conversos* (Jews who had converted to Christianity, been converted, or whose ancestors were thought to have converted) were seen as tainted and tainting. Whether Jews or Muslims (or imagined as such), whether Indians or Blacks, they were not real Christians: their blood was not pure. Shylock would soon hear about it, barred as he was from touching, much less sharing in, this new and extraordinary liquid: 'Christian blood'.

There is no doubt a universal dimension to blood. Yet, like many universals, this one has been produced and extended to those who would never have thought of bringing together for themselves blood and community, blood *as* community. It was a (slowly developing) Christian idea all along. And it has become a commonplace of anthropology, a discourse and discipline that is still fighting with its Christian inheritance ('systems of consanguinity', 'blood and belief'). More important for us here, blood has become Jewish, another 'rumour about the Jews' and a Jewish obsession. Such becoming started (badly) as an assignation and an accusation. It ended (worse) in doctrines of racial purity along the law and science to allegedly prove it. But we have never been Jewish. Not by blood.

FURTHER READING

- Gil Anidjar, ***Blood: A Critique of Christianity*** (Columbia University Press, 2014)
- David Biale, ***Blood and Belief: The Circulation of a Symbol Between Jews and Christians*** (University of California Press, 2007)
- Mitchell B. Hart (ed.), ***Jewish Blood: Reality and Metaphor in History, Religion, and Culture*** (Routledge, 2009)
- Carolyn Walker Bynum, ***Wonderful Blood: Theology and Practice in Late Medieval Northern Germany and Beyond*** (University of Pennsylvania Press, 2007)

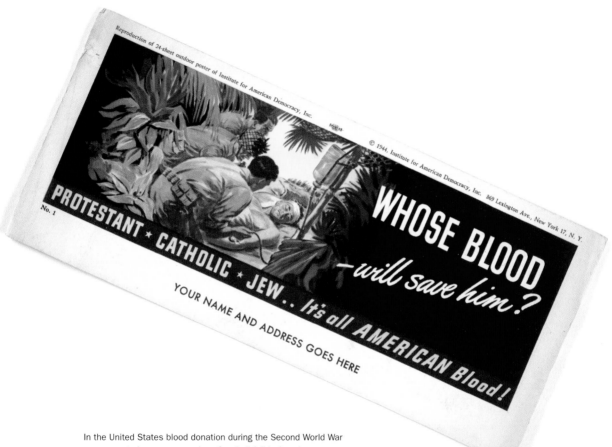

In the United States blood donation during the Second World War
was promoted as an expression of an indivisible American
citizenship. At the same time, however, the Red Cross separated
'Negro' from 'White' blood.
Jewish Museum London.

Orlando's Blood:
Red Thread Drawing
Jacqueline Nicholls, Artist

This is one of a series of embroideries that trace the movements of performers, using red thread as a symbolic replacement for blood. It takes the spontaneous drawings sketched during a performance and retraces and makes deliberate each line.

The Mishnah in Sanhedrin 4:2, which discusses the unique value of individual human lives, quotes the story of Cain killing Abel, describing Abel's bloods as screaming from the ground. The blood takes the place of the individual and demands justice. The usage of the plural 'bloods' has been interpreted to mean that Cain also killed all of Abel's potential – not just one life. Elsewhere in the Torah, when it is obligating us to take care and protect life, it uses the word 'blood' to represent the potential victim (for example, don't stand idly by the blood of your neighbour).

My grandmother always insisted that we had some red ribbon or thread attached to our clothes, as an amulet against the evil eye. By wearing the amulet of the red thread we are sending out a message that blood flows in this body, and this life should be protected.

© Jacqueline Nicholls

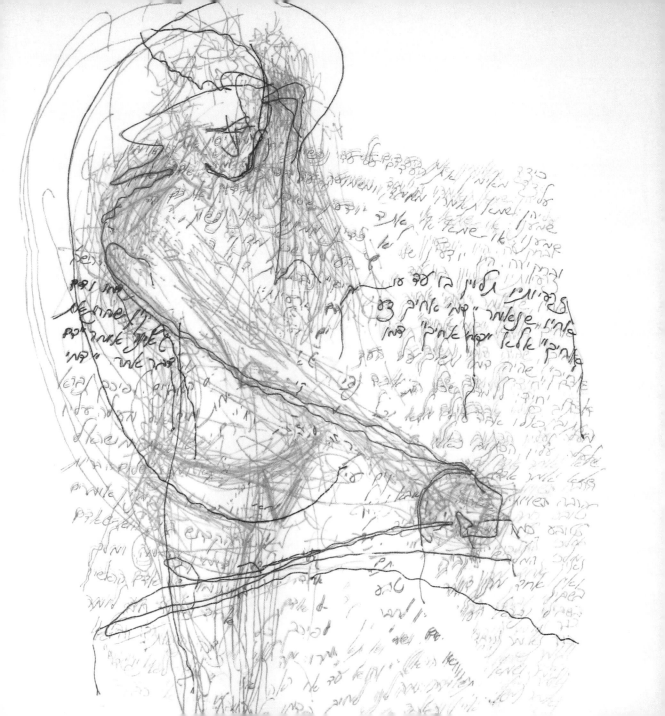

About the Authors

Gil Anidjar is Professor in the Department of Religion, the Department of Middle Eastern, South Asian, and African Studies, and the Institute for Comparative Literature and Society at Columbia University, New York. He is the author of, among others, *The Jew, the Arab: A History of the Enemy* (Stanford University Press, 2003) and *Semites: Race, Religion, Literature* (Stanford University Press, 2008).

Anthony Bale is Professor of Medieval Studies at Birkbeck, University of London. He has published two books on relations between Christians and Jews in medieval culture: *The Jew in the Medieval Book: English Antisemitisms 1350–1500* (Cambridge University Press, 2006) and *Feeling Persecuted: Christians, Jews, and Images of Violence in the Middles Age*s (Reaktion, 2010). He is currently researching pilgrimage, literature, and popular religion in late medieval Palestine.

Marc Michael Epstein holds the Mattie M. Paschall (1899) and Norman Davis Chair in Religion and Visual Culture at Vassar College and was Vassar's first Director of Jewish Studies. Professor Epstein has written on various topics in visual and material culture produced by, for, and about Jews, including *The Medieval Haggadah: Art, Narrative, and Religious Imagination* (Yale University Press, 2011) and *Skies of Parchment, Seas of Ink: Jewish Manuscript Illumination* (Princeton, 2015).

David Feldman is Director of the Pears Institute for the study of Antisemitism and also a Professor of History at Birkbeck, University of London. He has published widely on relations between Jews and non-Jews in modern Britain, as well as on the history of immigrants and ethnic minorities.

His books include *Englishmen and Jews: Social Relations and Political Culture, 1840–1914* (Yale University Press, 1994). He is currently researching the history of opposition to antisemitism.

Sander L. Gilman is Professor of the Liberal Arts and Sciences as well as Professor of Psychiatry at Emory University. A cultural and literary historian, he is the author or editor of over eighty books, most recently, *Illness and Image: Case Studies in the Medical Humanities* (Transaction Publishers, 2015); and the edited volume, *Judaism, Christianity, and Islam: Collaboration and Conflict in the Age of Diaspora* (Hong Kong University Press, 2014).

Robin Judd is Associate Professor of History at The Ohio State University and an associate member of the University's Melton Center for Jewish Studies. Judd is the author of *Contested Rituals: Circumcision, Kosher Butchering, and Jewish Political Life in Germany, 1843–1933* (Cornell University Press, 2007) and has published a number of articles concerning Jewish history, gender history, and ritual behaviour.

Dorothy Porter is Professor of the History of Health Sciences at the University of California San Francisco. She has published extensively on the history of public health, social medicine and genetics and eugenics, including *Health Citizenship: Essays on Social Medicine and Bio-medical Politics* (University of California Press, 2012) and *Health, Civilisation and the State: A History of Public Health from Ancient to Modern Times* (Routledge, 1999).